I Ate It, Now What?
Food, and its Journey Through your Body

By

Stanley W. Morey, Ph.D

Table of Contents

Acknowledgments

This book would have not been possible without the help of my wife, Gery Morey who helped me through organizing the chapters, and suggesting the explanation of many words that appear in the text. The suggestion for the title came from a great friend named Frank James who we call FJ.
My Granddaughters, Sarah Morey and Heather Morey as well as two of my friends, Robby Robinson, Masters Mr. Olympia, and Dr. Richard Baldwin, a Professor at Gulf Coast State College provided the inspiration for this book. I also wish to thank Liz Lamagese for converting my files into a usable format.

Introduction

Have you ever wondered what happens to the bite of your Hamburger once it enters your mouth? Well, it makes a miraculous journey through your Digestive System, and we will attempt to go through this magical process. I will explore this journey by describing what occurs to your food, from its initial breakdown, to its eventual absorption and elimination.

I will define Carbohydrates, Proteins, and Fats as well as Vitamins and Minerals, and the role of Enzymes and Herbs.

I will provide you with an intelligent way to analyze Diets, as well as to improve your Health. I will not offer you a miracle, or diet revolution, but a sensible way to analyze your food, which can lead to a healthier way of life.

Dr. Stanley W. Morey

Chapter 1. Foods, Vitamins, and Enzymes

Food? What is it? What does it do? The word food is taken for granted. Everyone assumes to know what food is, what a carbohydrate, protein, or fat is and what they do in relation to other food. However, in actuality, most people know very little about it. This chapter will thoroughly define the term food and its accessory substances: water, inorganic minerals, derived from non-living sources and organic matter derived from living sources.

In order for a substance to be termed a food it must accomplish certain things that will differentiate it from other substances entering the body. A food, or nutrient, must supply energy to the individual without causing damage. A perfect example of a non-food is alcohol, which provides energy but with side effects that are not beneficial. Food must also increase the amount of protoplasm, the essential living material in an organism that the body needs for growth or maintenance. And food must be able to be stored in the body for cases of emergency use and as a reserve supply of energy. There are three principal food groups: proteins, fats, and carbohydrates and they provide the body with energy and building materials. These food groups are also known as organic compounds because they all contain carbon. The body also requires water, mineral salts, and vitamins to enable it to utilize the organic compounds and only a combination of all of these substances will meet the requirements for growth and development.

A. Food
1. Water

People tend to overlook water but this simple compound, H_2O, is essential to life and without it we would be unable to exist. Our water intake is dependent upon the water contained in our food. Water, the universal solvent, serves many purposes and can dissolve many substances that then may pass quickly into the bloodstream. It also maintains the osmotic pressure (pressure required for moving things through a membrane) necessary for this passage, and is the fluid medium in which all chemical reactions occur. Some chemical reactions require water for their completion. Hydrolysis, for example, is a chemical addition of water to large molecules, which then splits them into smaller units. Water also plays an important role in the maintenance of body temperature, and is warmed as it passes through active tissues and then released as sweat. Plasma, the fluid part of the blood, is approximately 29 percent water, and combined with sweat is largely responsible for lowering body temperature.

2. Inorganic Minerals

Inorganic minerals (derived from non-living sources) are substances that are important in the regulation of cellular functions for two reasons (1) they exert their own osmotic pressure and are able to take part in the chemical reactions of the body (Table 1 lists these substances and some of their functions) (2) They are so vital to life that any major change in their normal levels is life threatening.

TABLE 1: INORGANIC MINERALS

ELEMENT	CHEMICAL DESIGNATION	BIOLOGICAL EFFECTS	EXCELLENT SOURCES
CALCIUM	Ca^{++}	Building of bones and teeth: aids in blood clotting, regulation of heart, nerve, and muscle activity, enzyme formation and milk production.	Asparagus, beans, cheese, cauliflower, cream, milk, egg yolk.
CHLORINE	Cl^-	Regulation of osmotic pressure, and enzyme activities; formation of hydrochloric acid in stomach	Bread, butter-milk, clams, cabbage, cheese, eggs, ham, table salt.
COBALT	Co^+	Normal appetite and growth; prevention of a type of anemia; prevention of muscular atrophy.	Liver, sweetbreads, seafood.
COPPER	Cu^{++}	Formation of hemoglobin; tissue respiration.	Bran, liver, mushrooms, oysters, peas, pecans, shrimp.
IODINE	$I, I-$	Formation of Thyroxin, regulation of basal metabolism.	Broccoli, fish, oysters, iodized salt, shrimp.
IR0N	Fe^{++}	Formation of hemoglobin; aids in tissue respiration.	Almonds, beans, egg yolk, meat, heart, kidney, liver, soy beans, whole wheat.
MAGNESIUM	Mg^+	Muscular activity, enzyme activity, nerve maintenance, bone structure.	Beans, bran, corn, brussel sprouts, peanuts, peas, spinach, prunes.
MANGANESE	Mn^{++}	Activates several enzymes; related to the utilization of vitamins B and E.	Brains, cheese, eggs.
PHOSPHORUS	**P**	Tooth and bone formation; buffer effect in blood; essential constituent of cells; muscle contraction.	Beans, cheese, eggs, liver, peas, oatmeal, whole wheat.

3. Organic Nutrients

Organic nutrients (compounds derived from living sources) serve as the principal source of energy and protoplasm formation. The three organic nutrients are carbohydrates, lipids, and proteins. The carbohydrates are the simplest in structure, lipids (fats and oils) are more complex and proteins are the most complex. These nutrients become constituents of protoplasm and give it those characteristics that make it different from all other known substances.

a. Carbohydrates

Carbohydrates are chemical compounds composed of the elements carbon, hydrogen, and oxygen (hydrogen and oxygen are present in a two to one ratio), and are divided into sugars and polysaccharides (poly=many; saccharide=sugar). The relative sweetness of some of the common sugars compared to sucrose, table sugar, can be seen in Table 2. (Not all sugars are sweet; in fact some are objectionable to the taste.)

TABLE 2: RELATIVE SWEETNESS OF SUGARS

Fructose (fruit sugar)	173.3
Glucose	74.3
Maltose	32.5
Galactose	32.1
Lactose (milk sugar)	16.0

*Optimal Nutrition, Coe and Morey 1979

The monosaccharides (mono=single) made up of six carbon sugars or hexose's (hex=six), are the simplest carbohydrates that can meet the energy needs of the body, their molecular formula ($C_6 H_{12} O_6$) is the basic structure of the carbohydrate used in human nutrition. The three principal hexose's in our diet that form the basis of our sugar metabolism are glucose, fructose, and galactose.

The disaccharides (two-sugar units) are a more complex group of carbohydrates. Green plants manufacture these during photosynthesis, a process that chemically combines the hexose's. When any of these disaccharides is present in the diet, it is broken down into hexose's by hydrolysis.

The polysaccharides are the most complex of the carbohydrates (starch contains almost 1,000 hexose groups) and, like disaccharides, must be broken down into monosaccharide units before the body can use them. The most common polysaccharides are glycogen (stored in animals), starch (stored in plants), and cellulose (structural material in plants). The carbohydrates serve many important functions in the chemistry of our bodies. Their oxidation quickly releases large amounts of energy; consequently, carbohydrates are stored in almost all tissues of the body (except the brain). The largest storage areas are the liver (glucose is carried by the blood to the liver where it is converted into glycogen for storage). In a normal, well-nourished individual, glycogen may account for almost 20 percent of the dry weight of the liver.) Muscles and kidneys also contain a sizeable quantity. Carbohydrates can also be converted into fats and stored. Hence individuals who overindulge may become overweight.

b. Lipids

The term lipid encompasses fats, which are solid at room temperature (20 degrees Centigrade), oils, which are liquid at room temperature, waxes and other fat-like substances present in many foods. Some lipids contain nitrogen and can supplement the proteins in forming protoplasm.

Chemically, the lipids are grouped into three subdivisions: (1) Fats and oils (2) phospholipids, and (3) Steroids.

Fats and oils can be subdivided into two groups dependent upon the amount of hydrogen present. (The molecule of a fat or oil, like carbohydrates, contains only the elements carbon, hydrogen, and oxygen; yet its structure is quite different.) Fats and oils that have many hydrogen bonds are termed saturated fatty acids and those with a smaller number of bonds are termed unsaturated. Unsaturated fatty acids can be converted to saturated by a chemical reaction with hydrogen called hydrogenation. (This is done commercially in the manufacturing of certain shortenings and butter substitutes, and usually makes them solid at room temperature.)

Fats are broken down to glycerol and fatty acids by the digestive process. Most of this digested fat is oxidized to produce energy; the rest is carried to the cells and stored as fat. The body stores fat chiefly in the food vacuoles, which are spaces or cavities within the protoplasm of a cell, containing nutritive or waste substances. Most of the adipose tissue in the body is thought to come from fat and carbohydrates. Primarily the fats in our diet contain many types of fatty acids. These acids all have characteristic and distinctive flavors and the mixture of acids gives foods their particular flavor and odor. The liver plays an important role in fat metabolism. It synthesizes fatty acids from carbohydrates, rebuilds fatty acids into characteristic human lipids, and oxidizes fatty acids in the process of making cholesterol, phospholipids or carbon dioxide and water. Lipotropics (affinity for fat) are necessary for the synthesis of phospholipids in the liver. Without them fat accumulates in liver cells and phospholipid formation is impaired. Three important lipotropics are **choline, inositol, and methionine.**

Humans require only small amounts of fat soluble vitamins and certain unsaturated fatty acids for optimal growth and maintenance, and outside of these, fat is apparently not essential in the diet. This indicates that all other fats can be synthesized from other nutrients at a rate adequate for normal growth and health.

It has been recognized for a long time that overweight people are more prone to cardiovascular disease than those who do not eat fat producing foods in excess. Fats are the most concentrated source of energy, yielding per gram over twice as many calories as carbohydrates or proteins. It has also been observed that in countries where the average diet is quite high in fats, the number of deaths from cardiovascular disease is greater than in countries where the diet contains little fat.

The phospholipids are a group of chemically complex substances containing nitrogen and phosphorus in addition to the carbon, hydrogen, and oxygen present in the fats and oils. They are abundant in the brain, kidney, heart, eggs, and soybeans. Lecithin is the best known Phospholipid, a normal constituent of cells. Egg yolk is particularly rich in lecithin and a crude preparation of lecithin can be obtained from that source.

Steroids are represented by cholesterol, the best-known member of this group. Cholesterol is found in great quantities in the brain and spinal cord, and has an important role in the formation of bile by the liver. In some individuals the cholesterol in the liver is converted into hard bodies, or gallstones, and these can cause serious difficulties if they obstruct the flow of bile.

Cholesterol has been given considerable publicity because of its role in one of the most common types of cardiovascular disease. Deposits of cholesterol may form in the walls of the coronary arteries, which supply the heart with blood. These deposits roughen the walls and encourage blood clot formation that may result in coronary thrombosis. The body's supply of cholesterol is not obtained solely from the diet since various body tissues synthesize it. However, there is evidence that the presence of large amounts of saturated fatty acids and sugar in our diet may be responsible for the formation of these excess cholesterol deposits. General weakening of the arteries may also occur due to cholesterol and calcium deposits the walls.

c. Proteins

Proteins, some of the most chemically complex organic compounds, have extremely high molecular weights and large molecular structures. They are composed of smaller units (amino acids) that are relatively simple. Forty amino acids have been discovered so far. However, only about 23 have been accepted as common "building blocks" and only 20 of these are widely distributed. No one protein has been found, thus far, that contains all of these amino acids, but casein of milk contains 18 of them. (See Table 3.)

TABLE 3: AMINO ACID CONTENT OF SOME PROTEINS
(Percent Dry Weight)

ESSENTIAL	GELATIN	CASEIN	EGG WHITE
Arginine	8.0	4.3	6.0
Histidine	0.8	2.9	2.9
Isoleucine	1.3	6.4	7.0
Leucine	2.9	7.9	9.9
Lysine	4.1	8.9	6.5
Methionine	0.9	2.5	5.3
Phenylalanine	2.6	4.6	7.2
Threonine	2.2	4.9	4.0
Tryptophane	-------	1.6	1.2
Valine	2.3	6.3	8.8

NON-ESSENTIAL	GELATIN	CASEIN	EGG WHITE
Alamine	10.0	3.8	7.6
Aspartic Acid	7.5	8.4	9.3
Cystine	0.1	0.4	2.8
Glutamic Acid	10.8	22.5	16.5
Glycine	26.0	2.3	3.8
Proline	16.5	7.5	3.8
Serine	3.4	6.3	8.2
Tyrosine	0.4	8.1	4.1

Proteins vary in structure according to their source. The proteins in one tissue of an animal's body will differ from those found in another tissue. These differences depend on the number and type of amino acids present, their ratio by weight and number, and their arrangements within the protein molecule. Amino acids are also divided into two groups. Those that are essential amino acids (which must be supplied by the diet), and those that are non-essential amino acids. There are 10 essential amino acids that must be present in the diet because the body either cannot synthesize them or does so too slowly. The non-essential amino acids can be synthesized out of other materials in our food and are just as important as the essentials for proper body growth and maintenance.
The primary function of dietary protein is to repair and replace protoplasm and to form new living material. Nitrogen is the essential element in the protein molecule and without it protoplasm could not be produced. It is interesting to note that although the

element nitrogen composes about 80 percent of our atmosphere we are unable to utilize it for protoplasm formation.

A second function of dietary protein is to supply energy. There is some question as to whether proteins are oxidized directly for energy or first converted into sugars and fats. If they are oxidized directly, their production of energy is equivalent to an equal amount of carbohydrates.

The fuel value of each of the classes of organic nutrients, in terms of the heat produced when oxidized in the body, is as follows:

1 gram of Carbohydrates	**4.1 calories**
1 gram of Fat	**9.3 calories**
1 gram of Protein	**4.1 calories**

Although carbohydrates and fats can be stored in the body, if they are in excess of caloric requirements, there is no provision for the storage of protein. Proteins that are not immediately utilized in the formation of new protoplasm are then built into the protoplasm of existing cells or are transformed into sugars and fats. Therefore, it is imperative that an adequate amount of protein be consumed in the daily diet to avoid negative nitrogen balance, a condition in which the body oxidizes its own tissues.

If you're in the market for a particular protein supplement, shop very carefully; never purchase protein by percent, which serves as a great advertising tool. For example, out of a package of 100 percent protein manufactured from a material high in indigestible fiber, we would be able to assimilate only a very small amount. A protein should be purchased according to its ingredients and/or Protein Efficiency Ratio; (the protein Product must contain the essential amino acids to be of best use.) The P.E.R. is a ratio of efficiency compared to casein, which is given a P.E.R. number of one. Numbers greater than one are more efficient; numbers below one are less efficient than casein.

The best ingredients to look for in a protein are (listed in order of efficiency) egg, milk and egg, milk-soy and egg, glandular, calcium caseinate, sodium caseinate, and soy-vegetable proteins.

B. Vitamins

The body's requirement for certain food factors has been known for many years. However, it has only been in this century that we have isolated and related these factors to specific body conditions. One of the first observations that specific factors were involved in disease states came forth in the sixteenth century. A British sailor, Richard Hawkins, noted that lemons and oranges prevented scurvy among his sailors. (However, it was almost 200 years later that James Lind, a British physician, recommended that the Royal Navy be given regular rations of limejuice.) In 1882 Admiral Takaki of the Japanese navy, in an attempt to relieve his men of the disease beriberi, increased the rations of meat, barley, and fruit, alas, to no avail. Dutch physician, Eijkman, five years later, discovered that a disease similar to beriberi could be induced in birds fed on polished rice; he later cured the birds by feeding them the husks of the rice that had been removed in the polishing process. He hypothesized that the lack of some factor present in the husks but missing from the polished grain might be the cause of the illness. His work stimulated the interest of physiologists and intensified their research in the field of food deficiency diseases. In 1911, Dr. Casimir Funk proposed a theory to account for these diseases. He gave those missing food factors the name *vitamine* because his work indicated that they all contained the amino (NH_2) group, which is characteristic of all amines. Later studies indicated that this was not entirely correct, so the spelling was changed to *vitamin*.

Vitamins are now known as essential food substances even though they don't actually contribute any material to the production of energy or protoplasm. They are only required in small amounts but without them the body cannot use some of the foods it takes in and could not carry on the numerous vital functions that are necessary for the maintenance of normal conditions. All of the known vitamins fall into one of two categories: those that are fat-soluble and those that are water-soluble. This difference is of considerable importance because it indicates how vitamins will behave in the body, when foods are cooked.

1. Fat Soluble Vitamins

The fat-soluble vitamins require the presence of bile in the intestinal tract for absorption; therefore, any defect in fat absorption may lead to deficiencies.

a. Vitamin A

Vitamin A, ($C_{20}H_{29}OH$) itself is not found in plants and is entirely a product of animal metabolism. It is a slightly yellowish substance that is stable when exposed to air at ordinary temperatures, but is rapidly destroyed in the presence of oxygen at high temperatures. (This explains why foods cooked in open pans usually lacked vitamin A while those prepared in pressure cookers retain it.) Our bodies convert a plant product, carotene, into vitamin A. (Three different chemical forms of carotene are found in plants. One of these can be converted into two molecules of vitamin A while the others produce only one molecule each.) Carotenes are yellowish in color and give the typical color to carrots and other plant foods. Cryptoxanthin, another yellow pigment, is found in corn and can also serve as a source of vitamin A. If large amounts of carotene are eaten the person's skin may take on a yellow discoloration and form excess freckles. Individuals who have a normal, adequate diet can store enough vitamin A in their liver to meet their needs for several weeks or months, should their supply be cut off. Retention of vitamin A, however, is apparently dependent on the presence of a second vitamin, vitamin E. Animals deprived of vitamin E are unable to properly store vitamin A because it is changed by oxidation. (Vitamin E is an anti-oxidant and prevents this change.) Vitamin A is essential to the health and well being of epithelial tissues (membranous or boundary tissues) and makes them less susceptible to disease. Since the lining of the digestive and respiratory tracts (as well as many glands) is made up of epithelium, the normal function of these organs is upset if vitamin A is lacking. If vitamin A is deficient, the tissue become dry and cells slough off. Glands do not produce their normal secretions. The secretions of tears may be lessened and the outer layers of the eye become dry and opaque. This condition is known as Xerophthalmia (dry-eye) and is a cause of blindness. Vitamin A is also essential for the proper formation of rhodopsin (visual pigment) in the rods of the retina of the eye. If vitamin A is partially lacking recovery from glare is slow and the ability to see in dim lights is impaired.

The proper formation of tooth enamel too, is dependent on vitamin A. If there is a deficiency in a child's diet, or in the diet of the mother before the birth of the child, the enamel is not properly formed. Pits may result in the surface of the enamel that may lead to early tooth decay.

The common foods that are rich in vitamin A contain a large amount of carotene (i.e.) all yellow vegetables and the outer leaves of cabbage and lettuce. Many leafy vegetables are also rich in carotene although the yellow color may be hidden by the green chlorophyll i.e., spinach, kale, collard and mustard greens. Animal foods, such as whole milk, butter, eggs, liver, kidney, and some fish are good sources of vitamin A.

b. Vitamin D

Vitamin D promotes the proper growth and development of bones and teeth and other structures when the mineral calcium is present. (There are two principal chemical forms of vitamin D, ($C_{28}H_{44}O$) and ($C_{27}H_{44}O$) and both are of equal value to humans.)

Vitamin D promotes the absorption of calcium and phosphorus from food, as well as improves the reabsorption of phosphorus in the kidneys. If it is lacking, rickets may develop even in a diet that contains adequate amounts of required minerals.

Human skin normally contains a sterol compound, cholesterol, and there is definite evidence that cholesterol can be converted by a series of complex chemical reactions into another compound, 7-dehydrocholesterol. This new compound is then converted into vitamin D_3 ($C_{27}H_{44}O$), by exposure to certain wavelengths of ultraviolet radiation. (Not all such radiations are capable of this conversion, some merely cause sunburns.) Another substance, ergosterol, which was first isolated in the fungus from which ergot is obtained, can also be converted into a vitamin D by ultraviolet irradiation. This is vitamin D_2 ($C_{28}H_{44}O$), which is produced in commercial quantities from yeast.

Very few foods contain significant amounts of vitamin D. Dairy products and eggs vary in their amounts depending on the exposure of the cows and hens to sunlight. It is possible, however, to increase the vitamin D content of these foods by feeding the vitamin to the animals. Milk may also have its vitamin D content increased by exposure to ultraviolet radiations. Since vitamin D, like vitamin A, is stored in the liver oils pressed from the livers of cod, halibut, and shark is a commercially important source. Salt-water fish, such as herring, mackerel, salmon, and sardines contain relatively large amounts of vitamin D. Vitamin D deficiency appears to be common because of the use of sunscreens and other methods used to prevent sunburn. Exposure to the sun only a very short time daily can correct this problem.

c. Vitamin E

Another group of fat-soluble vitamins is vitamin E. Chemically, these vitamins belong to the group of organic compounds known as tocopherols, a name derived from the Greek words tocos (child birth) and phero (to carry), because they are necessary for normal reproduction. There are six different tocopherols that have approximately the same effect, but one, alpha tocopherol ($C_{29}H_{50}O_2$), are the most potent.

Vitamin E prevents fats from oxidizing and becoming rancid. (This antioxidation effect makes vitamin E necessary for the proper use and storage of vitamin A, making it essential in the stability of tissues.) The tissues of vitamin E deficient animals, particularly cardiac and skeletal muscle, consume oxygen more rapidly than do normal tissues, implying that vitamin E is necessary for the proper function of these tissues. The richest sources of vitamin E are plant oils (wheat germ, rice, and cottonseed) as well as the lipids of green leaves. Vitamin E supplementation is common, however, it is not necessary in most cases.

d. Vitamin K

There are two naturally occurring forms of vitamin K: K_1 ($C_3H_{46}O_2$) and K_2 ($C_{41}H_{56}O_2$). Vitamin K_1 is present in food while Vitamin K_2 is normally formed in the intestinal tract by bacteria. Both can be absorbed only if bile is present in normal quantities. In addition to these, there are several synthetic, water-soluble forms of Vitamin K. Vitamin K_3, or menadione, is more effective than the oil-soluble form since it can be absorbed by the blood stream directly at locations other than the lacteals (walls of the intestines). Vitamin K is involved in the blood clotting mechanism. People taking Warfarin and/or Coumadin make occasionally have to have vitamin K injections when their clotting mechanism becomes hazardous.

TABLE 4: OIL-SOLUBLE VITAMINS

ELEMENT OR VITAMIN	CHEMICAL DESIGNATION	BIOLOGICAL EFFECT	EXCELLENT SOURCES
A	$C_{20}H_{29}OH$	Vitamin A is essential to the health and well-being of the skin, bones, teeth, gums, and hair.	Yellow vegetables, kale, spinach, collard and mustard greens, whole milk, butter, eggs, liver, kidney, and some fish.
D	$C_{28}H_{44}O$ $C_{27}H_{44}O$	The "sunshine vitamin" helps the body to absorb and utilize calcium, phosphorous, and other essential minerals. Vitamin D not only maintains bones and teeth but is vital to the metabolic functions that directly affect the heart and nervous system.	Saltwater fish, such as herring, mackerel, and salmon, contain relatively large amounts of vitamin D. Sunshine
E	Tocopherols $C_{29}H_{50}O_2$ (alpha–tocopherol)	This essential oil-soluble vitamin is present in all body tissues where it plays critical roles with red blood cells.	Plain oils, wheat germ, rice, and cottonseed, as well as green leaf lipids.
K	K_1 - $C_{31}H_{46}O_2$ K_2 – $C_{41}H_{56}O_2$	Involved in the blood clotting mechanism.	Pork.

2. Water Soluble Vitamins

B-complex vitamins - In the early days of vitamin research a substance was discovered that prevented beriberi in humans. Later work in the field has shown that what was originally thought to be a single substance is actually a group of compounds, which we now call vitamin B complex. B complex is necessary for the formation of many enzymes particularly those involved in energy reactions and the formation of red blood cells.

a. Vitamin B1, Thiamine Hydrochloride

Vitamin B_1, ($C_{12}H_{17}CLN_4OS$ HCL) is also known as the antineuritic vitamin because its inclusion in the diet will help prevent the appearance of certain types of nervous disorders. If birds are kept on a thiamine deficient diet partial paralysis of their muscles, polyneuritis, will result. In humans, there is a retardation of growth, loss of appetite, degeneration of the nervous system, muscular difficulties, enlargement of the heart, and eventually death.

A person's ability to absorb and use this vitamin properly is important. Increased intake of thiamine may be required to offset the effects of diarrhea.

Thiamine is often used in cases of severe gastrointestinal disorders or extensive surgery of the digestive tract. Occasionally, beriberi has appeared in people who suffer from tuberculosis, dysentery, or cancer of the liver. Chronic alcoholism may lead to beriberi because the diet of a heavy drinker is usually low in thiamine. **The process of polishing grain, white rice and white flour removes thiamine and the use of these products should be avoided.**

Thiamine forms a phosphate salt, a coenzyme known as cocarboxylase, within the cells. This coenzyme is essential for complete oxidation of carbohydrates to carbon dioxide and water, the normal end products. In its absence, various intermediate substances accumulate (i.e. pyruvic acid) and upset the metabolism of cells. Since the brain derives its energy almost exclusively from the oxidation of carbohydrates, any disturbances in the oxidation of these compounds makes itself evident in abnormal function of the nerve cells of the brain. Very little thiamine is stored in the body. Some small amounts are normally present in the liver, kidneys, and muscles but these are quickly metabolized. Bacteria in the intestine may be able to synthesize thiamin but not in sufficient quantities to satisfy the body's needs. Thiamine is found in many foods. Its richest sources are the husks of grains, wheat germ, milk, potatoes, cabbage, meat (especially pork), eggs, and brewers yeast. It is easily destroyed by heat. In dry heat there may be a loss of from 10 to 25 percent and cooking in water the loss may be as great as 50 percent.

b. Vitamin B2, G-Riboflavin

Riboflavin, ($C_{17} H_{20} N_4 O_6$), is a yellow compound that is stable in air and dry heat but easily destroyed by light and is widely distributed in foods. It aids in the release of energy from cells, and also regulates some vital activities. It is able to form members of a group of substances known as flavo-protein enzymes. These belong to a large group of enzymes, the oxidases that are active agents in releasing energy within the cells. Riboflavin may also play a role in vision. It is present in the pigment of the retina of the eye, where it aids in light adaptation. A deficiency of riboflavin results in retarded growth in some experimental animals. In humans, a lack of riboflavin causes sores on/around the lips and mouth, scaly skin, increased sensitivity of the eyes to bright light, and the growth of fine blood vessels over the surface of the eyes, which eventually leads to blindness.

c. Vitamin B3, Niacin (Nicotinic Acid), Niacinamide (Nicotinamide)

Vitamin B_3 is a constituent of two coenzymes that play vital roles (oxidation-reduction reactions) in metabolism. Niacin is also a strong vasodilator, which causes a flushing of the skin (niacinamide does not cause flushing). Niacin also maintains normal gastro-intestinal function and is involved in the proper functioning of the nervous system. Additionally, niacin is involved in the metabolism of carbohydrates. In large doses, about 1 gram given three times daily, niacin appears to lower serum cholesterol level (a physician should be consulted). Niacin is removed in most milling operations of grains.

However, it can be made from the amino acid tryptophane, which remains. Deficiency may result in dermatitis, diarrhea, and in acute cases, pellagra. Good sources of niacin include liver, poultry, and milk.

d. Vitamin B5, Pantothenic Acid

Pantothenic acid, ($C_9 H_{17} O_5 N$), has an important role in cellular metabolism. It is a constituent of the compound called coenzyme A that is essential in the formation and breakdown of fatty acids and the liberation of energy from fats and carbohydrates. Also, it is required for the formation of hemoglobin and various sterols, such as cholesterol, and some of the reproductive hormones (steroids). Brewers yeast, liver, and royal jelly are good sources of pantothenic acid.

e. Vitamin B6, Pyridoxal, Pyridoxamine, Pyridoxine

In common with some of the other vitamins, vitamin B_6 plays a role in cellular metabolism. It was noted in a study of rats that had been kept on a B_6 deficient diet that there was a pronounced failure of some of the sulfur containing amino acids, such as tryptophan, to function properly. If this condition were permitted to continue, recovery would be impossible, even if B_6 were to be given to the rats. In humans, especially infants who are fed on a highly artificial diet, the most apparent symptom of the lack of vitamin B_6 is cerebral seizures resembling epilepsy.

Experiments using healthy, human volunteers who were kept on a diet deficient in vitamin B_6 produced changes in the encephalogram (EEG) patterns. The onset of this condition was hastened by reducing the protein intake of the subjects. These experiments indicated a direct connection between the presence of vitamin B_6 and the proper utilization of proteins in tissues, especially those of the central nervous system. B_6 is also involved in fatty acid metabolism; however, the exact process is obscure. In large quantities, vitamin B_6 may act as a diuretic. The amount of dietary B_6 required is unknown; some B_6 is supplied to the body by the activity of intestinal bacteria. The National Research Council has recommended 1-2 mg per day. However, recent studies indicate that this is not entirely sufficient and that supplementation might be necessary. B_6 is abundant in milk, fresh vegetables, whole wheat, and much meat. It is not easily destroyed by dry heat but is destroyed by moist heat and will readily dissolve when food is cooked in water.

f. Vitamin B12, Cyanocobalamine

Vitamin B_{12}, ($C_{63} H_{90} N_{14} O_{13} PCo$), in its pure form is a red crystalline compound that is not affected by heat in a neutral solution, but is rapidly destroyed by heating in acids or alkalis. It contains the element cobalt (CO), an infrequent constituent of protoplasm. The discovery of the action of vitamin B_{12} required careful detective work. It was known that folic acid helped in the treatment of pernicious anemia, but did not actually cure the disease. Further investigation showed that an extract of fresh liver could be used to treat pernicious anemia. Also, it was found that victims of this disease improved after treatment with an extract of muscle tissue plus normal gastric juice. However, gastric juice from a person ill with pernicious anemia was not effective in this treatment. These facts indicated that two necessary factors must be present. Careful chemical analysis of muscle and liver tissue indicated that both tissues contained B_{12}, the so-called extrinsic factor. Normal gastric juice contains the intrinsic factor, whose function is to assure the proper absorption of vitamin B_{12}. Vitamin B_{12} is normally formed in sufficient quantities by bacteria in the large intestine. As coenzyme B_{12} it takes part in synthetic reactions in conjunction with folic acid. B_{12} is also involved in nucleic acid metabolism, formation of red blood cells, and growth mechanisms. Good sources of vitamin B_{12} are liver and kidney. Moderate amounts can be obtained from milk, lean meats, and fish. It is found in very low concentrations in plant products, an important factor for vegetarians.

g. Folic acid, Folacin (Pteroylglutamic Acid)

The primary role of folic acid, ($C_{19} H_{19} N_7 O_6$), is believed to be nucleoprotein synthesis. It is also important in mammalian cells during mitosis (cell division). Its relationship to B_{12} is close but unclear, but they are both (B_{12} & Folic Acid) involved in hematopoiesis (blood cell formation). Folic acid may be synthesized in the intestine and is concerned with the use of proteins for growth and development. Folic acid and biotin are required for the proper utilization of pantothenic acid. Good sources of folic acid are liver, kidney, mushrooms, and yeast.

h. Inositol

Its use is still vague; however, its presence in large quantities in the heart, brain, and skeletal muscle precludes its necessity as a food supplement. It may act in the utilization of CO_2 in certain chemical reactions in the cell. Inositol is also involved in fat metabolism in the liver (lipotropic). Inositol is widely distributed in plant and animal cells.

i. Biotin, vitamin H

The exact relation of vitamin H, ($C_{10} H_{16} O_3 N_2 S$), to human nutrition is not well understood. Recently, however, it has been shown to play an important role in fatty acid synthesis. If rats are kept on a biotin-free diet they develop a severe itching of the skin. Then the hair around their eyes falls out (spectacle eye) and eventually baldness results. In humans, skin changes, weight loss, and muscle pain have been ascribed to lack of biotin.

A biotin-free diet contains raw egg white as the principal source of protein. Raw egg white contains an enzyme, avidin, which combines with biotin and makes it unusable by the body.

RAW EGG WHITE (AVIDIN) + BIOTIN = STABLE COMPOUND NOT ABSORBED

Cooking destroys the avidin, as well as rapid blending. Although biotin may not function like some of the other vitamins in regulating a definite process, it plays an important role in the body's chemistry. It appears to be an essential part of a coenzyme that is required to form citrulline, a substance that is necessary for the production of urea by the liver. Biotin has recently been implicated in proper hair growth and balding. Biotin is present in greatest quantities in liver, yeast, and poultry. Some bacteria in the liver intestine can synthesize it.

j. Choline

Choline, although not considered a true vitamin, plays an essential role in nutrition. Choline is a constituent of the lecithins and is directly involved in fat metabolism (lipotropic). Choline can be synthesized from the amino acid methionine. In the forms of acetylcholine it acts as a mediator of nerve activity. Choline is widely distributed in glandular tissues, egg yolk, and a few vegetables. Its deficiency causes tissue damage and the abnormal accumulation of fat particularly in the liver, and also in the heart and blood vessels.

k. PABA, ParaminoBenzoic Acid

Very little factual information is available on PABA; however, it is involved in melanin production and can serve as an excellent sunscreen. It has been implicated in growth processes and steroid production but this link is still rather uncertain.

l. Vitamin C, Ascorbic Acid

Vitamin C, ($C_6 H_8 O_6$) is now commonly known as either antiscorbutic vitamin or ascorbic acid. The former name is used because this vitamin acts as a specific agent in the prevention and cure of scurvy. For many years this disease was prevalent among sailors and explorers who were deprived of fresh fruits and vegetables for long periods of time. Strangely enough, farmers have shown some signs of scurvy when relying on home-canned vegetables. When vegetables are prepared for home canning by boiling them in open pots, vitamin C is destroyed. If such vegetables are used to the exclusion of fresh ones, the symptoms of scurvy appear.

The absence of vitamin C from the diet will result in fragility of the capillaries and subsequent loss of blood. This condition is due to a weakening of the cement material that holds the endothelial (tissue of blood vessels and lymphatic tissues) cells together. Tooth structure may also suffer from improper formation and maintenance of the dentine. Also, the cementum that holds the tooth in its body sockets weakens and the tooth becomes loose. These effects are accompanied by a loss in weight and constant and annoying pain in the joints. Extreme deficiency of vitamin C may sometimes result in death.

The amount of ascorbic acid required by pregnant and lactating women is considerably higher than at other times. This increased requirement is due to the demands made on the mother by the unborn child for enough vitamin C to build skeletal structures and maintain a normal condition of the blood vessels. Also, an increase of vitamin C appears necessary following severe injury or surgery. It has been found in these cases that the amount of ascorbic acid in the serum of the blood decreases and it becomes concentrated in the scar tissue that forms at the wound site. An inadequate amount of vitamin C slows the healing process. This relationship is due to the action of the vitamin in speeding up the formation of collagen fibers. These elongated fibers of protein form the basis of connective tissues, and its formation will be slowed or stopped in the absence of vitamin C. A process that is accelerated by the presence of an adequate amount of ascorbic acid is the absorption of iron through the intestinal walls. Research has shown that certain types of nutritional anemias can be improved by the addition of extra vitamin C to the diet. The adrenal cortex contains large quantities of vitamin C, which suggests its uses in the synthesis of steroid hormones. This vitamin evidently plays a number of roles in cellular metabolism that are not all clearly understood at present. Some of these are associated with the utilization of the amino acid tyrosine. Humans, unlike most animals, have no method of synthesizing vitamin C and depend on their diet for their supply; nor do they have the capacity to remain in a healthy condition if deprived of vitamin C for a long period of time. Thus a liberal daily intake of vitamin C, throughout life is recommended.

Vitamin C is the least resistant of the vitamins; heating and drying usually destroy it. It is sensitive to oxidation, which is hastened by contact with metals, such as iron and copper. There is also considerable loss of vitamin C during storage, canning, and cooking. Vitamin C is found in large quantities in fresh tomatoes, turnips, green leafy vegetables, and the majority of fruits. Fresh meats contain Vitamin C in moderate amounts.

Table 5. WATER-SOLUBLE VITAMINS

ELEMENT OR VITAMIN	CHEMICAL DESIGNATION	BIOLOGICAL EFFECT	EXCELLENT SOURCES
B_1	Thiamine hydrochloride	Helps create energy from food by promoting the proper metabolism of carbohydrates.	Husks of grains, wheat germ, milk, potatoes, cabbage, meat, eggs, brewers yeast.
B_2	Riboflavin	Involved in the body's use of fats, carbohydrates and proteins particularly to help increase energy in the cells.	Widely distributed in foods.
B_3	Niacin, nicotinic acid, niacinamide	Present in all body tissues and is involved in the energy producing reactions within body cells.	Liver, poultry, milk.
B_5	Pantothenic acid	Necessary in body metabolism in converting fats, carbohydrates, and proteins into molecular forms needed by the body. Required in the formation of certain hormones.	Liver, brewers yeast.
B_6	Pyridoxine, Pyridoxal, Pyridoxamine	Performs many important roles in protein metabolism and in the use of fats. Also aids in the formation of red blood cells.	Milk, fresh vegetables, whole wheat, meat.
B_{12}	Cyanocobalamin	Helps in the building of nucleic acids for cell nuclei and in red blood cell formation. Aids in proper functioning of the nervous system.	Liver, kidney, milk, lean meats, and fish.
Inositol	-----	Involved in fat metabolism in the liver. Found in many tissues.	Widely distributed in foods.
Folic acid	Folacin, Pteoylglutanic acid	Assists in the formation of certain body proteins and genetic material for cell nuclei. Also helps in the formation of red blood cells.	Liver, kidney, mushrooms, brewers yeast.
Biotin	Vitamin H	Works throughout many of the metabolic systems. It participates in life-sustaining biological functions, such as carbohydrate, fatty acid, and protein metabolism.	Liver, brewers yeast, poultry.
Choline	----------	Functions in the metabolism of fats and in the prevention of fat build-up in the heart, liver, and other organs.	Glandular tissues, egg yolk, lecithin.
PABA	Paraminobenzoic acid	Melanin production. Excellent sunscreen. Aids in the growth processes and in steroid production.	Widely distributed in foods.
Vitamin C*	Ascorbic acid	Since the body does not manufacture Vitamin C, adequate amounts must be obtained every day from the diet or through supplementation. One major function is maintaining collagen, a protein needed for the formation of connective tissue. Also aids in the absorption and utilization of iron.	Fresh tomatoes, turnips, green leafy vegetables, and the majority of fruits. Fresh meats contain moderate amounts.

Heating and drying destroys Vitamin C, which is sensitive to contact with metals such as iron and copper. There is also considerable loss during storage, canning, drying, and cooking.

3. Enzymes

The growth and activity of every cell in the body is dependent on the presence of a group of chemical compounds, known as the enzymes. The chemical activities of enzymes are so varied and complex that they accomplish with ease processes that a chemist can reproduce only with difficulty. (An enzyme is a complex compound capable of being involved in a chemical reaction without itself being changed in composition. The chemical name for this is organic catalyst.)

The outstanding characteristic of an enzyme is its ability to accelerate chemical change without entering into the reaction. This can be likened to the action of a drop of oil beneath a metal weight on an inclined glass plate. The oil does not start the weight moving down the plate, nor does it combine chemically with either the metal or the glass, it merely speeds up the sliding process. Thus far all enzymes that have been isolated and chemically identified are proteins. In many instances these proteins cannot function by themselves but require the presence of some other substances (co-factors). Some of these accessory materials are relatively simple, like calcium or magnesium ions, while others are highly complex.

We have learned that vitamins are very important for the human body. However, we have also learned how fragile they can be. Heat, the materials they are cooked in, and the canning process easily destroys some of theses vitamins. We should be able to get all the vitamins we need from our food, but because of refining, cooking and processing most if not all vitamins are destroyed or made ineffective. The result is that we probably need to supplement these vitamins. However, we need to be very careful that the products we choose meet FDA requirements, and even USP certification.

Chapter 2. Digestion and Assimilation

In the last chapter we described what our food is likely to contain, such as Water, Carbohydrates, Proteins, Lipids and Enzymes. We will now discuss the journey our food will take during the Digestive process.

Food begins its amazing journey in the mouth, and continues on its voyage as it is digested and absorbed, and finally removed as waste.

Join us now as we begin this amazing journey.

A. Digestion in the Mouth

Enzymes bring about chemical digestion in the alimentary tract. These enzymes are classified as follows: 1) sugar splitting enzymes, the glucosidases that hydrolyze disaccharide's to monosaccharides; 2) amylolytic or starch splitting enzymes, such as salivary amylase and pancreatic amylase; 3) lipolytic or fat splitting enzymes, such as lipase; 4) proteolytic or protein splitting enzymes, such as pepsin, trypsin, and chymotrypsin. The process of digestion actually begins by cooking. In the process of cooking, starches are broken down to dextrins, fats to glycerol and fatty acids, proteins are hydrolyzed to a certain degree and bacteria and parasites are killed.

Digestive processes are divided into mechanical and chemical. Mechanical digestion includes the various physical processes that occur in the alimentary canal. These processes serve the following purposes:

    1. Taking in food, and moving it along the digestive tract at the optimum rate.

    2. Lubricating food.

    3. Liquefying.

    4. Grinding.

The following terms are used to define these processes:

    1. Mastication: breaking down and mixing with saliva.

    2. Deglutition: swallowing.

    3. Peristalsis: keep things moving.

    4. Defecation: bowel movement.

Chemical digestion is essentially a process of hydrolysis (decomposition in which a compound is split into other compounds by taking up the elements of water) dependent on the presence of enzymes. Chemical digestion is necessary to break foods down into their assimilable or usable forms.

The mouth is the first part of the digestive system with which food comes in contact. The sight and smell of food stimulate the nervous system, which in turn stimulates the body to dilate the blood vessels in the mouth, causing the salivary glands to secret a large amount of watery saliva. (This is called the psychic phase.)   When food enters the mouth the nervous system constricts the blood vessels in the mouth, and the salivary and buccal glands produce a thicker secretion of saliva. This causes the digestion of starch by salivary amylase into dextrins and maltose. Absorption in the Mouth is quite good, we should chew our food thoroughly for maximum assimilation.

B. Digestion in the Stomach

Food that enters the stomach is reduced into a thin liquid, called chyme, by the process of peristalsis. Gastric juice provides an acidic medium (pH. 0.9 - 1.7), and is produced in quantities of 1.5 to 2.5 liters per day. A normal meal will remain in the stomach for a period of 3 to 4 hours.

Gastric juice is composed of the following:

Hydrochloric Acid (HCL). HCL activates pepsinogen and converts it to pepsin. HCL provides the acid medium in which pepsin is active and swells protein fibers, thus increasing their surface area. HCL also breaks down sucrose and is an antiseptic.

Pepsin. Pepsin is a weak proteolytic enzyme requiring an acid medium for optimum action. Pepsin initiates protein digestion (breaking protein particles down into smaller molecules).

Rennin. Rennin is present only in infants and young adults. It has a strong action on casein, the protein of milk. One part of this enzyme is able to convert 4,500,000 parts of milk into a curd in approximately 10 minutes at a temperature of 40 degrees C and a ph value of 6.2 (Pepsin 1: 800,000). The fact that the ph value of the adult stomach is considerably below that necessary for the proper digestion of milk is a strong argument against its presence in adult digestive systems. We are probably one of the few animals that use milk after we are weaned.

Gastric lipase. Another stomach enzyme about which there has been much debate among physiologists is gastric lipase. It has the ability to break fats down into fatty acids and glycerol. There appears to be a small amount of this enzyme formed in the stomach, but its action is very weak because it is destroyed when the acidity of the stomach becomes higher than 0.2 percent. The extent to which it affects fat is unknown, but any action it might have would occur early in the digestive process and in connection with the breakdown of fats, like those found in milk and ice cream.

C. Digestion in the Small Intestine

The chyme produced in the stomach enters the small intestine at the duodenum. It is normally free of coarse particles, and is acidic due to the hydrochloric acid and lactic acid produced during fermentation. Much of the food entering the small intestine is undigested (Proteins have only been partially hydrolyzed, some starch digestion has occurred, and fats have been liquefied) and most of the digestive process and assimilation will occur in the small intestine.

The peristaltic movement of the intestines, the pancreatic fluid, the succus entericus (secretion of the intestine) and bile bring about the digestive changes in the small intestine. The pancreatic fluid consists of a nervous system stimulated secretion and a chemical secretion. The nervous secretion is thick and red containing enzymes and proteins. The chemical secretion is thin and watery, contains few enzymes or proteins, and is alkaline in nature. The fluid contains three groups of enzymes: trypsin, which is involved in protein digestion, amylase, which is involved in carbohydrate digestion, and lipase, which is involved in fat digestion.

The intestinal secretion of succus entericus is a clear, yellowish fluid with a marked alkaline reaction.   The succus entericus contains the following enzymes:

1. Enterokinase: activates the enzyme trypsin.
2. Erepsin: hydrolyzes small chain proteins (peptides to amino acids).
3. Maltase: hydrolyzes maltose and dextrin to simple sugars.
4. Invertase: hydrolyzes sucrose to glucose and fructose.
5. Lactase: hydrolyzes lactose to glucose and galactose.
    In black adults, 80+ percent do not have this enzyme.
6. Nuclease: hydrolyzes nucleoprotein and also contains a hormone called secretin.

Bile is formed by the liver and is essentially a sodium bicarbonate solution. It consists of water, bile pigments, bile acids and salts, cholesterol, lecithin, and neutral fats. Bile enters the duodenum only during the period of digestion and between these times it is stored in the gall bladder. Mixtures of bile and pancreatic lipase digest fat more rapidly and bile is necessary for the absorption of fats. Bile is 1) a digestive secretion essential for the action of lipase; 2) an excretion of the liver that is responsible for removing toxins, metals etc. 3) an antiseptic.

D. Digestion in the Large Intestine

Food begins entering the large intestine within two to five hours after ingestion. Secretions of the large intestine contain large amounts of mucin and are alkaline. The intestinal flora (bacteria) in the large intestine brings about putrefaction of whatever proteins are still present. The intestinal flora synthesizes several B vitamins and vitamin K. Feces are formed here and defecation ensues. It normally takes a total of 20-36 hours for complete digestion in the alimentary tract. Unfortunately because of our refined foods, and the reduction of fiber in our diet this process takes a much longer time.

E. Digestion and Fiber

Dietary fiber is extremely important in any discussion concerning digestion or health. The term fiber, as it relates to diet, encompasses a group of carbohydrates including lignin, cellulose, pectin, and hemicellulose. Only plant foods carry these substances. One of the best and cheapest sources of dietary fiber is wheat bran. This bran is the exterior part of the whole-wheat kernel. Unfortunately, for western industrial society, this outer layer is removed from the grain kernel when it is processed into white (refined) flour. **That's why white flour is virtually devoid of dietary nutrients and fiber.** Since bran is approximately 85 percent dry material it will absorb up to nine times its own volume. For the individual who is on a weight loss program, large amounts of bran are very helpful. It gives the individual the feeling of being full with a very low amount of food. In addition, high fiber diets pass quickly along the large and small intestine. This rapidity of movement prohibits the absorption of additional calories through the intestinal wall that end up as stored energy (fats) around your waistline. Also, a study by Dr. Kenneth Heaton of Briston University has proved that bran actually prevents some absorption of calories, although how and why is not yet understood.

Chapter 3. Caloric Expenditure

A. Metabolism

Finally our food has completed its amazing journey through the digestive system, Nutrients have been broken down and absorbed, and waste materials have been eliminated.

The sum total of the chemical changes the body performs with its assimilated nutrients is termed Metabolism. In some metabolic changes large molecules are synthesized from smaller ones, for example, amino acids are put together to form proteins. These synthetic changes are termed **anabolic** and they create the materials needed for the body's structural and functional components.

In other metabolic changes, large molecules are broken down into smaller ones. For example, glycogen (a string of glucose molecules) breaks down into separate glucose molecules. These degradative processes are termed **catabolism.**

B. Basal Metabolism

Basal metabolism can be defined as the heat given off when physiological work is at a minimum (in the morning after a comfortable night's rest, relaxed in bed, or before breakfast). It should be obvious that any increase in physiological activity increases the metabolic rate over the minimum. The Basal Metabolic Rate is not the minimal metabolism necessary for mere maintenance of life, since there are times, (e.g., during sleep), when the metabolic rate may be lower than the basal rate. BMR is quite constant in individuals. However, many factors body size, age, sex, climatic conditions, diet, physical training, drugs, etc., may alter its rate.

TABLE 6. THE EFFECT OF MUSCULAR ACTIVITY ON BMR

ACTIVITY	PERCENT INCREASE IN BASAL RATE
Sleeping	-0.1
Working as draftsman	+54
Working as radio mechanic	131
Driving car	139
Dressing	242
Using pick to dig earth	498
Walking at 4.2 mph	678
Farming	712
Lumbering	1028
Walking in loose snow carrying 40 lb weight at 2.4 mph	1627
Weightlifting	2200
Typing at 40 wpm	51
Washing dishes	54
Sweeping	89
Carrying a tray	130
Changing bed linens	451
Skiing on level, hard snow, moderate speed	1002

Obviously size is an important part involved in influencing the Basal Metabolic Rate. There are four important factors involved in heat loss from the body: The temperature difference between the environment and the organism. The nature of the surface that radiates the heat. The area of that surface. The thermal conductance or the ability to absorb heat by the environment.

Surface area appears to be the most important of these factors. In fact, the basal metabolism of various mammals studied is roughly proportional to surface area. Normal BMR is about one calorie burned per hour for each kilogram of body weight. Another way to approximate BMR is to multiply one's weight, in pounds, by 10 (for women) or 11 (for men). **The usual BMR for adult women is between 1,200 to 1,400 calories per day, for men it's between 1,600 to 1,800 calories per day.**

Age and sex affect basal metabolism. The values are higher in childhood than in adult life and are uniformly higher in the male than in the female of the same age group. Heat production gradually declines with advancing age. Environmental temperature also appears to influence BMR. The basal metabolism of individuals living in a tropical climate is usually lower than the basal metabolism of similar individuals living in colder climates. Temperatures above 30 degrees C can cause a slight rise in the metabolic rate and body temperature. When the temperature falls below 15 degrees C, muscular tone increases, shivering may ensue, and heat production increases. Muscular training, as in athletes, may be reflected in a slightly elevated BMR. Certain drugs, e.g., epinephrine and thyroxin, will also cause an increase in BMR.

Food and muscular work may alter metabolism from the basal level. Caloric restriction may be accompanied by a considerable decline in total metabolism. Conversely, ingestion of food is followed by an increase in heat production above the normal basal level. (Of the three major foodstuffs, the ingestion of protein causes the greatest elevation in total metabolism.) The stimulating effect of food on the heat production of the organism is called the Specific Dynamic Action (SDA), which is the extra heat produced by the organism over and above the basal heat production as a result of food ingestion. In the case of protein, the specific dynamic effect amounts to approximately 30 percent; for carbohydrates, 6 percent; and for lipids, 4 percent, respectively, of the energy value of the food consumed. Therefore, it is essential in calculating the caloric value or equivalent of a diet to make provisions for the calories dissipated as heat resulting from SDA.

Muscles are capable of utilizing the energy of oxidation for the performance of mechanical work with an efficiency of approximately 30 percent. Moreover, when involved in hard work, the total energy required for performing this work may be many times that reflected by the BMR.

Mental effort produces little increase in metabolism. Studies have shown that the mental effort associated with the preparation for examinations or for solving mathematical problems led to an increase of only 3 or 4 percent in metabolism. Intense emotion may elevate metabolism 5 to 10 percent above the basal level.

C. Calories and Weight Control

Weight loss, weight gain, and weight maintenance have become mathematical computations. A gain or loss of 3,500 calories per week in the diet amounts to a gain or loss of one pound. If we also note that the average adult participating in moderate activity requires 15 calories per pound to maintain weight, it becomes very simple to calculate a dietary regimen for gaining, losing, or maintaining weight. Example: For a 200 lb. adult, the dietary prediction is as follows:

Maintenance: 3,000 cal/day
Lose 1 lb/wk: 2,500 cal/day
Gain 1 lb/wk: 3,500 cal/day

On any dietary program well-balanced meals should be consumed and junk food avoided.

D. Calories During the Growing Years

With growing children it is important to provide energy over and above that required for the internal workings of the body and muscular activity in order that additional nutrients may be available for development of body mass. During periods of rapid growth, the increased allowance should be as much as 10 percent. As growth rate declines, the allowances needed per unit of body weight decreases, even though the total food requirement is more because of the larger body mass.

It's during the growing years that proper eating habits must be established to provide the basis for a long life of health. Many parents are overly concerned about their active children not eating enough to "grow on." What parents should do is provide regular mealtimes, varied foods, a well-balanced diet, and freedom for the child to choose the amount of food he/she wishes so that they will develop good eating habits, and limit the risk of becoming overweight. With the American population now approaching 30 % obesity. It is very important to watch what we eat, and avoid fast foods.

E. Calories and the Athlete

Generally, caloric intake should not be severely restricted during the developmental period of an athlete's life. At the same time, an overweight growing athlete suffers a severe competitive handicap and should be advised to restrict caloric intake unless the increased physical activity alone will sufficiently bring about weight loss.

During the mature years when metabolism has slowed from adolescent years, nutrition for the athlete becomes more important. A well-balanced diet, including vitamin and mineral supplements to compensate for the reduction in caloric intake, should be followed.

F. Calories During Pregnancy and Lactation

The Food and Nutrition Board of the National Academy of Sciences (1980) considered an extra allowance of 300 calories per day sufficient for most women to meet their energy needs throughout pregnancy. Nursing mothers require an additional 500 calories per day during the first three months of lactation to provide for the caloric cost of producing milk. For the average mother who produces approximately 850 milliliters of milk per day, the caloric cost of lactation amounts to about 770 calories per day. For this reason, some nutritionists have recommended breast-feeding as a means of weight control in the overweight lactating mother. Another important fact is the production of Colostrum, which acts as an antibody during the first few days of lactation. A well-balanced diet and vitamin/mineral supplementation is also of prime importance for the health of the mother and the child.

Chapter 4. Diet and Deflabbing

When the subject of diet comes up in conversation it is always interesting to listen to the various methods employed to achieve the same basic goal - weight loss. There are so many "diets" available to choose from that one begins to wonder, do any of them actually work? And, if they do work, how? Adding to the general confusion over this subject is the lack of distinction by the public at large between a reduction of total body weight, and the elimination of excess body fat (which is generally found in the waist and buttock areas). When discussing "dieting" most people probably mean a combination of these two. The degree to which total weight and excess body fat merge, is directly dependent upon the progression of obesity. A person who is 50 pounds overweight will reduce total body weight to body fat in a greater ratio than a person who is five pounds overweight. In essence, then, "dieting" in today's connotation is in fact synonymous with deflabbing, a non-technical but exact description of losing fat.

A. Comparison of Diets

Generally, all of the more popular diets, if properly followed, will result in temporary weight loss. The key word here is **TEMPORARY.** Follow-up studies have found that over 90 percent of the people who begin a "diet" regain the weight lost within the first year. You might as well face the facts: There is no such thing as permanent weight reduction without changes in wrong eating habits. Additionally, all of the different diet plans, except the High Fiber Permanent Weight Loss Plan, have serious long-term medical consequences. This is because more and more studies are finding that low fiber in the American diet is one of the major causative factors in heart disease, arteriosclerotic disease, high excessive cholesterol levels, cancer of the colon, diverticular disease, varicose veins, and other serious health problems. Any diet that is not high in fiber content may result in your being the slimmest, trimmest corpse around. That is why I incessantly state that dieting cannot be safely understood unless it is placed within the context of overall health. (See Table 7.)

Therefore, we should try and understand the mechanics of how the body actually works, from the initial introduction of food to its final use as energy by the body.

TABLE 7. COMPARISON OF THREE BASIC DIETS

PREMISES

LOW-CARBOHYDRATE	LOW-PROTEIN	HIGH-FIBER
Obesity is caused by the ingestion of excess carbohydrates (over 60 grams), or by carbohydrate intolerance.	Animal protein is consumed in too great a quantity, is deleterious and contains too much saturated fat.	Lack of fiber is a deficiency state, which leads to obesity, constipation, and other digestive ailments. In addition, mounting evidence associates low-fiber diets with heart disease, colon cancer, and rectal cancer.

GOOD POINTS

LOW-CARBOHYDRATE EXAMPLE: ATKINS	LOW-PROTEIN EXAMPLE: PRITIKEN	HIGH-FIBER EXAMPLE: SIEGALS
Provides the dieter with a "satiated, full" feeling and it is effective in short-term weight loss. The diet is simple to follow since the American diet is basically a meat diet.	This diet eliminates meat, reduces fat consumption and contains adequate fiber. Weight loss Is good and energy levels remain high.	This diet is well-balanced, produces a "full" effect and eliminates the common digestive ailments prevalent in America. Weight loss is permanent and the diet is simple. Bowel movements will become regular, thus removing large amounts of fats, calories, and toxic waste before absorption.

FLAWS

LOW-CARBOHYDRATE	LOW-PROTEIN	HIGH-FIBER
This diet in the long run will produce ketosis (end product of fat metabolism) and acidosis. These will lead to irritability, dizziness, and headaches. The diet is also low in fiber and constipation could occur. Another flaw is to lump the consumption of refined carbohydrates, such as sugar, with the use of natural, nutritious whole-grains, vegetables, and fruits.	This diet eliminates some excellent protein foods such as fish, poultry, and eggs. The diet is also boring and it is time consuming to prepare the varied meals.	Initial production of gas, which is only temporary.

WEIGHT-LOSS RATING

LOW-CARBOHYDRATE	LOW-PROTEIN	HIGH-FIBER
Good	Good	Excellent

LONG-TERM USE

LOW-CARBOHYDRATE	LOW-PROTEIN	HIGH-FIBER
Poor (side-effects of ketosis, acidosis, irritability, etc.)	Good (difficult to prepare meals, uninteresting)	Excellent (ease of diet, coupled with permanent results)

B. Carbohydrate Machine

When we discuss the automobile, we all know its basic fuel is gasoline. The human body also has its basic fuel, the carbohydrates, or even more exact, the six-carbon sugars. Everything we eat eventually must be converted into a six-carbon sugar in order to provide energy. The process by which energy is produced is termed the Krebs Tricarboxylic Acid cycle.

Our total biochemical and physiological make-up is geared towards a high carbohydrate, moderate protein, and low fat diet. It has always been a mystery why so many varied and exotic diets have come and gone, when we only have to study our body chemistry to design a "balanced diet" based on those requirements.

The primates, gorillas, apes, monkeys, of which we are a part, do not include meat or animal protein as part of their diet. Yet, these animals remain fit and muscular on a basically fruit and vegetable diet. The answer, or course, is that they are (as we are) carbohydrate machines, geared to operate on carbohydrates as fuel, using protein and fat as structural and storage components of their diet.

C. Meat Myth

We have been duped in this country to believe that meat is the basis for a healthy, nutritious diet. We are known worldwide as the "meat and potatoes" country because of the tremendous amounts of meat consumed by our society. It is estimated that meat purchases by the average American family can account for as much as 40 percent of the average total weekly food costs.

Along with the consumption of meat and the reduction of grains and fruit from the diet comes obesity. The rate of obesity in our country is growing at an alarming rate. We actually accept as normal a 16 percent body fat composition for males and 26 percent body fat composition for females as normal. This would make European countries shudder.

Meat, especially red meat, should be a small part of the diet because of the following factors: Cost - meat is expensive. Calories - meat is an extremely high calorie food. Fats - meat contains high levels of fat, especially saturated fats. Fiber- meat has virtually no fiber. Digestibility- our bodies are not geared to digest meat as efficiently as other foodstuffs, thus leading to increased levels of stomach acidity. This acidity leads to heartburn and indigestion. Meat provides excess protein that cannot be utilized and is excreted. More importantly, meat contains virtually no carbohydrates.

D. Protein Myth

If meat were eliminated, where would we get our protein? Along with the consumption of meat we have also been led to believe that protein in large amounts is essential to our diets. In this country we consume tremendous amounts of protein. Meat has been advertised as the perfect protein. However, this is not true. Based on the Protein Efficiency Ratio (P.E.R.), meat ranks poorly next to egg and milk products. In fact, egg protein ranks high in P.E.R., digestibility, assimilation, and amino acid content, with milk following close behind. The cost of egg and milk protein is also considerably more economical than an equal amount of meat protein.

E. What About Cholesterol

Cholesterol is also a very important product in our lives since many of our hormones are manufactured from cholesterol. One of the biggest fears people have is of getting too much "cholesterol" in their diet. Eggs have been avoided because of the belief that high levels of cholesterol cause build-up and blockage of the blood vessels and eventual heart disease. But in reality, eggs contain large amounts of the lipotropics (affinity for fat), choline, inositol, and methionine that have been shown to keep cholesterol levels in balance.

Researchers are finding more and more hard evidence that it is not excess cholesterol that causes heart and arteriosclerotic disease, but rather the lack of a substance known as high-density lipoprotein (HDL). As this HDL is carried through the bloodstream it consumes unused cholesterol before arterial wall irritation and plaque build-up can occur. It has been found that small amounts of alcohol, onions, and garlic increase the HDL level. Drs. Edward Gruberg and Steven Raymond have additionally found that a deficiency of Vitamin B-6 may also be associated with heart disease and recommend 5 to 25 mg. a day.

Cholesterol is not solely obtained from the diet. Various body tissues also manufacture it. In fact, the amounts obtained in the diet are minuscule compared to the amounts produced by the body. There is some evidence, however, that the presence of large amounts of saturated fatty acids and refined sugars in our diet may be responsible for the formation of excess cholesterol deposits in the arteries.

F. The Role of Fiber

In the United States, cancer of the colon and rectum have become the number one killer (Reuben, 1975.) In fact, there are approximately 49,000 deaths per year or one death every 10 minutes from these cancers. Studies have shown that one of the biggest contributing factors in the development of these cancers is a lack of fiber in the diet. English researchers studying native Africans, who rarely contract any ailments such as cancer, diverticulosis, appendicitis, and constipation, found that Africans processed their food completely to bowel movement within 24 hours after ingestion and voided up to two pounds of stool per day. Whereas Englanders took three days to as long as two weeks to completely process their food and voided only four ounces of stool per day. It was concluded that the fiber in the Africans diet was the reason and they felt that roughage was an urgent requirement for our diets. In fact, they considered lack of fiber an actual deficiency state.

Before 1916, colon cancer, rectal cancer, and even heart disease were rare. The current rise in the occurrence of these diseases can be directly attributed to the milling of grains (removing the fiber or bran) and to the increased use of refined sugars. The rise in the use of refined sugars has also resulted in an increase in obesity, and though considered a common condition today, obesity was once thought of as a disease.

The alarming lack-of-fiber problem is easy to correct. Changes in diet or adding small amounts of inexpensive wheat or oat bran to food can increase fiber intake substantially. There is simply no excuse for Americans to be fiber deficient.

It has also been noted that a diet high in cereal fiber increases the excretion of cholesterol from the body thereby lowering high cholesterol levels in the body. In fact, high fiber diets reduce cholesterol even though the individual may be on a high fat diet.

To convert the average American diet to a high fiber diet would only require the following steps. 1) Using of whole-grain products, such as whole wheat, rolled oats, and brown rice.

2) Eating fresh fruits and vegetables, raw or barely cooked, with seeds, strings, and skins intact (if possible). 3) Cutting to a bare minimum refined sugars, soft drinks, saturated fats, and meat.

1. High Fiber and Obesity

Obesity in the United States is no longer mere fertile territory for comedians to harvest sarcastic jokes, nor is it only the rich person's boredom produced preoccupation with trite banalities of weight. It is fast becoming a national health disorder. The U.S. Public Health Department has estimated that up to 60 percent of the U.S. adult population is overweight with 50 percent of those being obese (obesity for males begin at 20 percent body fat and 30 percent body fat for females). After age 25 the average person will add one pound of excess weight for each year of life. Every pound of excess fat contains approximately 200 miles of capillaries that your heart must supply with blood. As a result of this extra burden the heart must function almost continually at full speed and literally will work itself to death. Consequently, it has been statistically found that a person decreases his/her longevity by 1 percent with each excess pound of weight. Thus, if a person is 50 pounds overweight, he/she has a 50 percent chance of dying prematurely. So, is it any wonder that coronary heart disease is responsible for one third of all the deaths in the United States? And why were obesity and heart disease virtually unheard of before the late 1800s/early 1900s?

The answers to these questions will explain why I stated earlier that diets other than the High Fiber Food Plan are an invitation to disaster.

2. High Fiber and Heart Disease

Did you know that the average adult American male over 45 has one chance in two of having a heart attack before reaching his 65th birthday? The good news is that a simple change in dietary eating habits can do more to prevent this dreaded disease than all the nitroglycerin tablets put together. The findings among medical researchers are now incontrovertible. The basic difference between those 700,000 individuals who succumb yearly to coronary thrombosis and those who don't is essentially diet.

To better understand heart disease and heart attacks, you must first have to understand how incredibly unique and strong this muscle is. A few facts amply demonstrate this point.

The Heart:
1. Weighs approximately 12 ounces.
2. Is about six inches long and four inches wide.
3. Has four chambers and two pumps – one sending blood to the lungs – the other sending blood to all other parts of the body.
4. Pumps blood through 60,000 miles of blood vessels daily (the average person who is of average weight).
5. Is the strongest muscle in the body except for the woman's uterus (during childbirth)
6. Generally requires 10 times the amount of nourishment required by other body.

Heart attacks occur when plaque from the arterial system breaks off and becomes lodged in one or more of the coronary arteries surrounding the heart (the blockage may be no larger than a piece of pencil lead). When this reduction occurs you have become a statistic and a victim of America's dietary madness.

3. High Fiber and Cholesterol

Most experts recognize that excess amounts of cholesterol are largely responsible for the arterial plaque deposits that eventually cause heart disease. That's why we hear so much about low cholesterol diets: if you lower the cholesterol level in the blood stream, you lower the chance of heart disease. However, this is not exactly correct. The body receives cholesterol from two different sources. First, the liver produces approximately 1,000 mg of cholesterol daily, while; second, the average American diet adds another 600 mg. Since many of our hormones are manufactured from cholesterol, it is essential that the body have this substance in the proper amounts. Scientists believe that even a severely restricted diet, one that eliminates virtually all foods with high amounts of cholesterol, is fruitless because the liver simply produces the additional cholesterol needed for body maintenance.

So cholesterol, in and of itself, is not dangerous but rather essential. Excess cholesterol is the culprit. But why has excess cholesterol become a problem only since the early 1900s? Most people would answer, incorrectly, that it is due to the increased amounts of foods containing high quantities of animal fats, such as eggs, butter, milk, and meat. The facts, however, are quite to the contrary.

Prior to the industrial revolution and the gradual redistribution of our population from the farm to the urban areas, Americans consumed far greater amounts of these products on a per capita basis than they do today. We must, then, look for other causes of this excessive build up of cholesterol.

A diet lacking in high fiber is the key to understanding this problem. We have seen that heart disease is the number one killer of American citizens. We have also seen that excess cholesterol is one of the major causative factors in these heart attacks. Additionally, we have found that this problem did not exist before the turn of the century. Let us now take one further step in understanding why excess cholesterol levels exist and why this is a recent phenomenon.

Studies have found that a diet high in fiber dramatically affects the body's cholesterol level in two very significant ways: 1) Fiber increases the amount of cholesterol eliminated in excrement and 2) fiber decreases the production of cholesterol by the liver. (I believe that this very point is the fulcrum upon which a correct understanding of the interrelationship between diet and an overall approach to health is best illustrated and why I do not believe that diet books, per se, are healthful or helpful.) But first let me explain how and why a high fiber diet plan does this.

Part of the cholesterol manufactured by the liver is converted into bile acids that are critical to the digestion process in general, and, more specifically, help aid in the breakdown of animal fats. After passing through the small and large intestines these bile acids eventually end up in the colon where they are attacked by massive amounts of bacteria. People who eat a low fiber diet have billions of antibile bacteria known as bacteroides and bifidobacteria that attack the harmless bile acids and convert them into, among other things, a substance known as *lithocholate.* This toxic substance prevents the liver from converting cholesterol into the bile acids. This in turn leads to excessive amounts of cholesterol accumulating in the bloodstream and becoming implanted in the arterial walls. Furthermore, since the excess cholesterol is not converted to bile acids it cannot progress to the colon where it can be eliminated. The significance of this cannot be underestimated since the primary method by which the body can dispose of the harmful amounts of cholesterol is through the evacuation of excrement. Hence, the unused amounts of cholesterol remain in the body's system. The resulting build up of this cholesterol over a period of years causes the gradual blocking of the arterial pathways leading to heart disease, heart attacks, and even death.

Conversely, individuals on a high fiber diet have billions of very helpful bacteria known as streptococcus and lactobacillus in their colon. Unlike their counterparts in the low fiber diet, these bacteria do not break down the bile acids into harmful substances, but are quickly eliminated in the bowel movement. This not only removes dangerous amounts of cholesterol from the bloodstream, but also does something else very interesting. It activates what I believe to be the body's own built in method of safely regulating the amount of cholesterol present so as to avoid dangerous levels; and it does this in the following manner:

A high fiber diet causes daily evacuation of excrement contained in the intestines and colon. Bile acids, which are converted from cholesterol, pass through the digestive system to elimination. Consequently, with regular and daily bowel movements, the body is compelled to continually convert large amounts of cholesterol to bile acids to replace these vital digestive fluids. Thus, the liver converts more and more cholesterol into harmless bile acids that require further conversions and so on. The only remaining cholesterol in the system is that which is required to properly carry out the necessary bodily functions and all of the excess cholesterol is converted to bile acid and eliminated via the daily bowel movement.

It seems transparently clear that the low fiber diet is primarily responsible for heart disease in this country. It also seems just as clear that a high fiber diet would help to curb the major cause of this dreaded reaper of American lives.

4. High Fiber and Cancer of the Colon

Our discussion of high fiber and cholesterol holds the key to understanding why heart disease and cancer of the colon are directly related to each other and that the common "denominator" of both of these problems is a lack of high fiber in the diet.

As previously stated, a low fiber diet results in the accumulation of billions of harmful bacteria identified as bacteroides and bifidobacteria. I also stated that this harmful bacterium breaks down the harmless bile acids into a substance known as lithocholate that, in effect, prohibits the liver from changing cholesterol into bile acids. These very bacteria that are dramatically involved in causing heart disease (America's No. 1 killer) are also just as responsible for cancer of the colon (America's No. 2 killer). The reason is that the harmful bacteria, in addition to breaking down the bile acids into lithocholate, cause the remainder of the acids to be changed into a known carcinogen, 3 methyl-cholanthrene. As we have seen, the low fiber diet does not provide for prompt evacuation of fecal matter, which in turn causes the bacteria in the colon to change from helpful to harmful. When this occurs it allows the harmless bile acids to be converted into the acknowledged cancer causing agents. The end result is that the colon becomes a virtual colony of lethal agents. And just think, what pain, suffering, and loss could be avoided by the simple addition of 24 grams of fiber in a person's daily eating habits.

5. High Fiber and Weight Loss

One of the most popular and incorrect dietary notions is that reducing carbohydrates is the answer to weight control. This type of dieting has been around for many years, under many names, and has been attractive to people because it promised to reduce hunger as well as weight. However, many medical authorities including the American Medical Association, have condemned this dietary practice as being potentially hazardous. The reduced carbohydrate diet attempts to eliminate most if not all carbohydrates from the menu. The reasoning behind this is that the average obese person usually eats as many as 300 grams of carbohydrates daily. Therefore, if the carbohydrates are eliminated the weight will come down. However, Africans may consume as many as 3,000 calories per day, including 600 grams of carbohydrates, without ever becoming obese. Consequently, carbohydrates must not be the problem; lack of fiber is.

A high fiber diet will aid in weight loss because of the following:

A high fiber diet is more difficult to eat. Items such as Brown Rice, raw vegetables, and raw fruit require more time and energy to chew and assimilate than other types of food. A person will tend to eat less on this diet.

A high fiber diet is bulkier than a low fiber diet and will fill you up quicker.

High fiber causes a greater production of saliva and gastric juices. This causes fiber to swell that in turn distends the stomach and gives a feeling of being full.

There is evidence that a high fiber diet actually impairs the ability of the small intestine to absorb calories. Therefore, you can actually eat more and absorb fewer calories.

More fat is excreted in each bowel movement on a high fiber diet.

High fiber eliminates constipation, the ban of all dieters.

A high fiber diet allows you to lose weight without starvation. The diet is one of abundant food rather than food restriction. Instead of starving your fat away you eat your fat away. The excess flab will be gradually disappearing with a feeling of deprivation.

A high fiber diet is a diet that you can stay on for life. It is not just a fad or passing fancy; it is the way humans were supposed to eat and it should become a way of life.

6. High Fiber and Diet

The high fiber diet is not a temporary diet, as other diets attempt to be. Rather it is a way of eating for life. This system will normalize your digestive tract instead of altering it, as other diets do. Its basic principle is to eliminate fiber deficiency and to make normal digestion possible. When your body is normalized, it will regulate its weight within a normal range.

Several noticeable effects of a high fiber diet are:

1. The intestinal bacteria will shift to a more favorable lactobacillus-streptococcus form that will produce normal fermentation (rather than abnormal fermentation that can occur with other diets).
2. Fats, fatty acids, and toxic wastes are eliminated in greater quantities with each bowel movement.
3. The rate of absorption of the food you consume will decline.
4. Blood levels of fat should decline.

REMEMBER:
Breakfast like a king
Lunch like a queen
Dinner like a pauper

CONCLUSION

We have followed our food from its delivery into the mouth, its eventual assimilation, and its elimination as waste. We have also discussed Metabolism, and ways that our metabolism can be adjusted and/or changed. We finally ended by comparing diets and providing you the reader with a method to analyze proposed diets. We hope that we have achieved the goal of informing you the reader about the miraculous journey our food must make, and its eventual assimilation.

About the Author

Stanley Morey, Ph.D. is an accomplished author, writing many books in the bodybuilding and nutrition areas. He received his B.S. from the University of Tampa, attended J. Hillis Miller Medical School in Gainesville, and the University of South Florida, in Tampa. He received his Ph. D. from the University of the Pacific in 1972 in Physiology.

He was also a competitive bodybuilder for many years, winning many local and regional competitions.

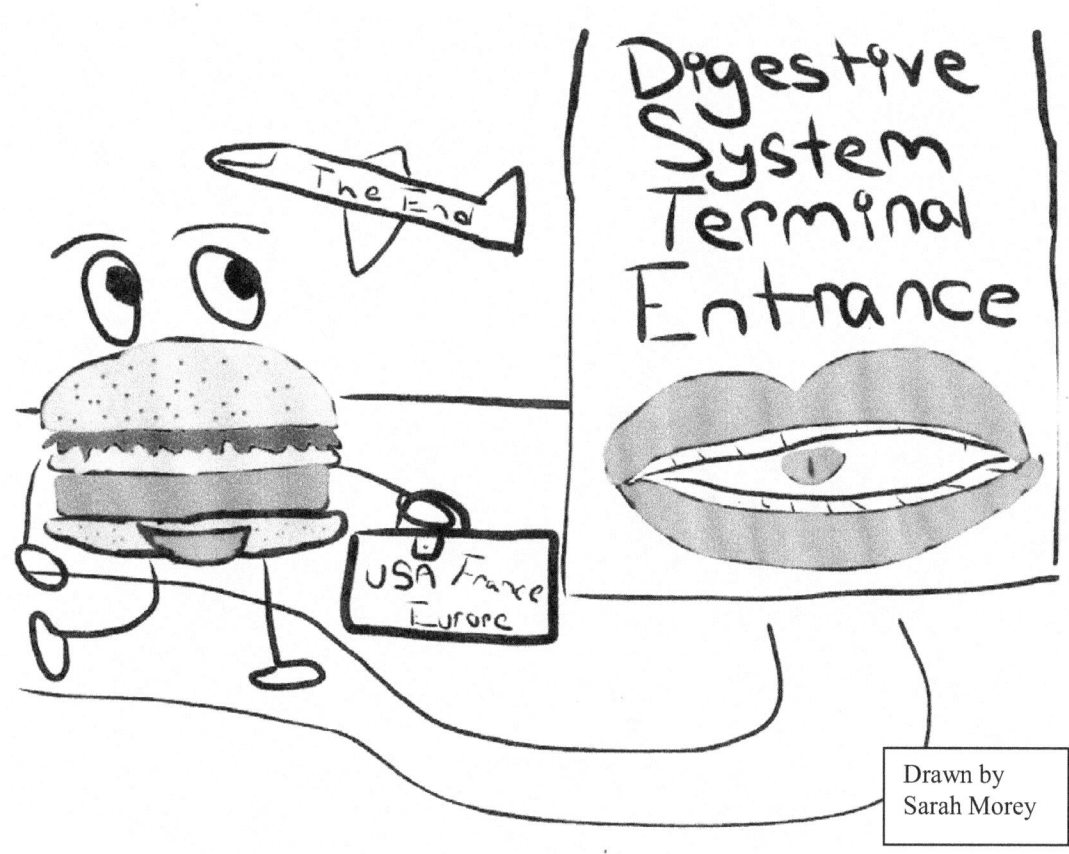

Drawn by
Sarah Morey